Run Yourself Skinny

The Beginner's Training Guide for Weight Loss

Jason Kayne

Table of Contents

INTRODUCTION

CHAPTER 1: THE BENEFITS OF RUNNING

CHAPTER 2: STARTING SLOWLY

CHAPTER 3: WHAT YOU NEED

CHAPTER 4: COMMON MISTAKES

CHAPTER 5: HYDRATION

CHAPTER 6: EATING AND RUNNING

CHAPTER 7: WEIGHT LOSS ADVICE

CHAPTER 8: HOW TO PREVENT INJURIES

CHAPTER 10: RUNNING WITH FRIENDS

CHAPTER 11: TRAINING PLAN

CHAPTER 12: HEALTHY FOODS FOR RUNNING

CONCLUSION

Introduction

Are you looking to lose weight? If you are like the majority of Americans, the answer to this question is a resounding yes. Some individuals only wish to lose five or ten pounds, yet others want to lose 100 pounds or more. Regardless of how much weight you wish to take off, running offers the best way to do so.

There are numerous benefits associated with running, but the key is to start slowly. You don't want to overdo it the first week or two and find you injure yourself or you become frustrated as you aren't seeing the desired progress. When you learn how to properly run, it's an enjoyable activity and one you can do anywhere.

When you start running, you want to have the right equipment. Most people assume any pair of shoes will do, yet this isn't the case. When you run, your feet take on additional body weight with each step you take. For this reason, you must ensure you have a good pair of running shoes. Once they have been purchased, however, you'll be ready to take off and start your training program.

Certain mistakes are made by many new runners. We'll cover these mistakes so you can avoid them and learn the right way to run immediately. Your diet plays a role in this, so you need to learn which foods will be of help to you before and after a workout, and you also need to ensure you stay hydrated. Both will help you to achieve success in this activity.

Preventing injuries is key, but you also want this activity to be fun and productive. With the help of weight loss advice, running tips and information on running with friends, you'll find everything you need to begin running today. Once you do, you'll likely be hooked for life.

Chapter 1: The Benefits of Running

Running offers numerous health benefits. Many individuals choose to take this activity up in an effort to lose weight. With running, you'll find you drop excess pounds and build muscle, and it only requires you run for 30 or 40 minutes three to four times a week.

With the loss of excess weight, your risk of heart disease, type 2 diabetes, liver problems and breathing issues decreases. Furthermore, running helps to reduce the risk of certain types of cancer, some forms of arthritis and osteoporosis. If you run consistently, you'll find your entire body benefits in both visible and non-visible ways.

The effects of running continue after you finish your workout for the day. This is known as afterburn, and studies have shown that the stimulation of afterburn is greater with running than with exercises of lower intensity. Resting energy remains elevated for a period of time after the run is over, and research shows running leads to 90 percent more weight loss than seen with walking.

Running is both convenient and time efficient. The only thing you need to run is a good pair of running shoes. This activity may be done anywhere, even when you are traveling, and it takes less time to run one mile than it does to walk, making this the perfect activity for those on a tight schedule. In fact, although many people now make use of short-intense workouts to burn more calories per minute, these workouts are so short, they don't offer the same level of caloric burn.

Another benefit of running is it helps to reduce symptoms of depression. Running releases a number of hormones in the body, including adrenaline, endorphins, growth hormones and insulin. Growth hormones and testosterone help with cell regeneration and muscle repair, while adrenaline and insulin convert fat into energy. The cortisol released as you run will reduce any stress you are experiencing and the endorphins boost your mood. They provide what many refer to as a runner's high.

Runners build endurance over time. If you find you are no longer able to do activities easily that you were able to in the past, such as playing with your children, running will provide you with more energy to do so. It takes very little time to notice an increase in your endurance. Often only a few weeks of consistent running will provide these benefits.

Chapter 2: Starting Slowly

Before starting any running program, visit a physician and have a complete checkup. Once you have done this, it's time to establish a running program. The first step tends to be the hardest, and a routine must be established. If you make running a priority and put it on your daily agenda, you'll find it is easier to stick with the plan.

Make certain to stretch after any workout, as stretching helps to reduce the risk of injury and prevents muscle shortening. If you feel you need to warm up before a run, start slowly and gradually build up speed. You don't want an injury to sideline you as you are getting started. You may be hesitant to pick back up when your injury is healed, for fear of being injured again.

Begin with a walking program. Walking places less stress on the bones and joints, yet allows the lower body to become more resilient and stronger. Some choose to combine walking and running the first few weeks, especially those who aren't overweight and are in fairly good shape. You may wish to do the same.

It's best to give the body a rest between running days, as this gives the muscles, bones and joints time to recover from the stress they have been placed under. Continue with the every other day program for several weeks. This does not mean rest days come with no exercise, as you may use these days for strength training or non-impact workouts, like walking or cycling.

Slowly increase the amount of time spent running. It's best to increase the distance of the run by only ten percent each week, as doing so helps to prevent injuries and/or exhaustion. Set a goal to reach 30 minutes of non-stop running and slowly work on this goal.

Consider joining a club, since most have groups for beginners, along with those who are more experienced. It's also a great way to find a running partner, someone to provide motivation when you are struggling. Ask around to find a club of this type or check with a local sports store. They may be able to assist you in locating a local running club.

Add variety to your running routine to keep it interesting. If you run the same route every day, you'll find you get tired of seeing the same sights over and over again. Try different routes, and run shorter distances some days and longer distances on others. Furthermore, take along some music or listen to an ebook. Consider checking into the beats per minute of your songs to ensure you aren't slowing down at times and picking up speed at others, and look for fast songs to keep you running at a good speed.

Chapter 3: What You Need

To run, all you need is a good pair of running shoes. You can run anywhere, in the city, on the beach or out in the woods. Your goal is to choose a pair of shoes that corresponds with the type of running you plan to do most often. Certain other factors should be considered, however, when purchasing a pair of shoes for this activity.

The only way to know if a pair of running shoes fits properly is to wear them on a run. Unfortunately, most stores won't let you try shoes for this long and then return them. For this reason, you need to make a few decisions before you head to the store to try shoes on.

As mentioned above, the first thing to consider when buying running shoes is where you plan to run. Trail-running shoes are designed for running off of the beaten path, places where rocks and other obstacles may be present. These shows have more tread to provide additional support, stability and protection for the foot. Road-running shoes allow you to run on pavement and other hard packed surfaces, those with only slight irregularities. They stabilize and cushion your feet as you run on these surfaces. Cross-training shoes, in contrast, are good for those who run as part of a gym workout, as they offer extra contact with the ground surface.

Once you have selected the type of shoe you need, you must look at how you run. If the inner part of your shoes show wear, you are more susceptible to knee pain and/or injuries, so you will need to purchase shoes that offer motion or stability control. If you notice more wear on the outer portion of the soles of your shoes, you need shoes that offer additional flexibility and cushioning. Very few runners have this type of wear pattern, however. Some runners do have neutral pronation, and this is biomechanically efficient running. Runners with this pattern will find they have more options when it comes to the shoes they choose, but most opt for a shoe offering moderate stability.

Know when to buy shoes for the best results, and take a pair of old running shoes along, as this helps to determine your wear pattern. Make sure you take the socks you wear when running to help find the right shoe fit, and buy in the late afternoon. Your feet are at their largest at this time, and your feet will expand as you run. Making a purchase at this time also helps to ensure the right fit. Don't purchase the latest shoe just because it looks good, because fit is more important in these shoes, and you'll want the salesperson to measure both feet also, as one foot tends to be bigger than the other. Finally, if you make use of orthotics, bring them when you shop for shoes. You need to ensure the shoe will fit with the orthotics in place.

Chapter 4: Common Mistakes

Make sure you set reasonable goals. You aren't going to get off the couch after being physically inactive for years and run a marathon the first week. It takes time to build up strength and endurance, so you will need to stick with the program for a period of time before you can do long distances. Don't get discouraged. With proper training, you'll reach your goal before you know it.

Never focus solely on running. Cross-training allows you to build different muscles in your body, so don't neglect your other training. Mix up your workouts, as this will help you to stay engaged and interested in running. In addition, doing so helps to prevent overuse injuries.

Make sure you are taking in enough calories. Although you are running to lose weight, restricting calories drastically can lead to stress fractures, as the bones weaken. In addition, if you aren't taking in enough food, you'll find it hard to build the muscle you want and need. Never try to lose more than two pounds in one week, and make sure you eat properly after a hard workout.

Don't let the arms hang down while running. Keep the arms naturally at the sides, while bending the elbows at 90 degrees. The elbows should move naturally back and forth at the waist and the fingers should be in a relaxed grip. Some runners allow the hands to sway back and forth in front of the torso. Don't do this, as it interferes with the natural running movement.

Pain is a sign your body needs to rest. Don't try to push through the pain, as this could do more harm than good. When you find you hurt, it's time for a break. Hurting is different than soreness or discomfort, so pay attention to what your body is telling you and take breaks as needed.

Chapter 5: Hydration

Hydration is of great importance when you run. You need to drink throughout the day, rather than just when you are running. The fluids you take in help to regulate your body temperature, while ensuring your joints are lubricated. They control cravings, so you'll find it is easier to lose weight, and the fluids help to remove waste from the body. In addition, water and other liquids work to flush out any cells that have become damaged. These cells can bring about inflammation that can interfere with your running.

Although the rule of thumb has always been to drink 64 ounces of fluid every day, runners often need more liquid. Drink a minimum of half of your body weight every day. A person who weighs 170 pounds should be drinking 85 ounces of water, and a person who weighs 200 pounds would need 100 ounces.

Fruits and vegetables are another great way to remain hydrated. Eat plenty of these foods when you run, and you'll find the risk of dehydration goes down significantly. Another benefit of eating fruits and vegetables is that they have plenty of antioxidants. This helps to boost your immunity while also helping in muscle recovery.

While running, continue to drink fluids, especially when you are running long distances. The key here is to drink to your thirst, as this helps to prevent over-hydrating. Under-hydrating tends to lead to dehydration, while over-hydrating can actually result in a low blood salt level, as your body retains too much fluid. For every 20 minutes you run, you should consume four to six ounces of fluid.

Don't hesitate to make use of sports drinks. A minimum of eight ounces is a good goal to aim for. This type of drink not only ensures a runner remains hydrated, but it also provides the potassium and sodium needed to have a healthy workout. One benefit of carrying a sports drink on a run is the electrolytes and carbohydrates found in these drinks help your body absorb the fluids faster.

Chapter 6: Eating and Running

A runner's diet affects their performance. Choose foods that will help you as your run, while trying to avoid empty calories. Eggs are great for runners, as they provide approximately ten percent of the protein you need every day. In fact, eggs fall only second to human breast milk in terms of their complete food protein. When you eat an egg, you will get the critical amino acids muscles need during the recovery process. Furthermore, you also get 30 percent of the recommended amount of vitamin K, a vitamin needed for healthy bones.

Carbs are also preferred before running. Try to consume items that are low in fat and fiber, and eat a minimum of 30 minutes before you run. After you finish your run, you should eat a snack high in protein to help with muscle tissue repair. Wait 20 minutes and then have this snack, but make sure it also contains carbs, as this will help to replenish the energy used.

Runners often struggle to meet their copper and manganese requirements, yet both are needed for the muscles to function properly. Although sweet potatoes only contain trace amounts of these nutrients, they also contain vitamin A, which is a robust antioxidant. Bake, boil or microwave them and watch your performance improve.

When you find you are lacking in energy, incorporate whole-grain pasta into your diet. The whole grains are not only easily digested, they also help to replenish your energy. Whole-grain versions will fill you up, thanks to their high fiber content, and this will help you to eat less and lose weight. As you go to choose a whole-grain pasta, look for one that contains B vitamins, as these vitamins aid in energy metabolism.

Muscle soreness bothers many runners, and eating oranges can reduce or eliminate this type of discomfort. When you eat an orange, you get more than 100 percent of the vitamin C you need each day. If oranges are eaten regularly, you'll find you aren't as sore after a good workout, and oranges provide numerous other benefits also.

If you struggle with exercise-induced asthma, add salmon to your diet. With the consumption of salmon, the inflammation response in your body is more balanced. As a result, you'll see a reduction in your asthma symptoms within a few weeks, but look for wild or farm-raised salmon to limit the risk of PCB or mercury contamination.

Consider eating an energy bar or fruit approximately two hours before tackling a run. Another great snack food you should stock up on is frozen mixed berries. They help you to recover after a run and promote muscle repair. Dark chocolate is great for when you want to indulge, because it helps to fight infection, a problem when you have an injury. It's also a great treat if you are struggling with a craving for sweets.

In Chapter 12 you will find a list of recommended healthy foods for runners.

Chapter 7: Weight Loss Advice

You didn't gain the weight overnight, so keep this in mind as you are trying to lose it. You aren't going to drop 20 pounds after running for only a month, unless you drastically reduce your caloric intake. Doing so does more harm than good, however, and can lead to health issues, such as stress fractures, as mentioned before.

This does not mean you can eat more, nevertheless. Many individuals find they aren't losing the desired weight, and the reason for this is they are eating more food because they are now running. You need to eat fewer calories than you are burning off if you wish to see progress. In addition to running, you may wish to track your caloric intake for a few weeks, to ensure you know how many calories you are taking in every day and how many you are burning off.

Challenge yourself. Not only will this help to keep you motivated, you'll find interval training or speed work can help you to burn more calories. If you use this technique, you will see a boost in your muscle mass and your resting metabolism improves. This means you burn more calories all day long, not just when you are working out. Only one interval session is needed each week to see additional weight loss.

Make sure you run consistently. You'll need to run at least three to four days a week to see weight loss. Try to run for a minimum of 40 minutes, because recent studies show doing so allows you to burn more calories per hour for the next 19 hours! Who doesn't like this?

Chapter 8: How to Prevent Injuries

Stress fractures are commonly seen in those who are new to running. To prevent this type of injury, you need to slowly build up your running distance and speed. If you find your pain gets worse when you exercise, but gets better when you rest, you may have a stress fracture. Make sure you get plenty of rest. If you continue to exercise with a stress fracture, you may find the injury becomes much worse, sidelining you for an extended period of time.

Muscle pulls are another problem many new runners struggle with. This is nothing more than a small tear in a muscle, and many call it a muscle strain. When you stretch a muscle too far, you'll find you have this problem. Many runners describe a popping sensation as the muscle tears. You'll need to rest the muscle, ice it down, use compression and elevate it as much as possible.

Achilles tendonitis is when the Achilles tendon becomes inflamed. This is the tendon that runs from the calf to the back of your heel. You'll find that this tendon is painful and stiff, especially when you are active or when you get up in the morning. This injury occurs when the tendon is put under repetitive stress and often occurs when you add too much distance to your runs too fast. Calf muscles that are tight also contribute to this problem. Do calf stretches, rest the tendon and ice it regularly to reduce pain in the area.

Sore knees and shin splints tend to plague many new runners. Immediately treat these issues with ice packs following a workout, and use a bag of frozen vegetables if nothing else is available. In the event the pain persists, rest for several days before resuming the training program. The body is saying it needs time to rest and heal, so listen to it.

Try to run on soft surfaces. A soft surface reduces the impact on your body, because you are transmitting less force to your bones and tendons. Never run on cambered gutters in roads either, as they can increase the amount your ankles roll inward and bring about Achilles tendonitis.

Chapter 9: Running Tips

Humidity can affect running. Try to run early in the morning or late at night during periods of high humidity. Don't hesitate to walk at various points in a run when the weather is hot and humid. In addition, make sure to cover up with sunglasses, sunscreen and a hat that keep the sun off the face.

Set a goal. The goal provides the motivation you need to stay engaged when you get discouraged. Many find training for a race is great for providing this motivation, but each runner needs to find the thing that works for them.

Occasionally take a break from running and make use of a cross-training workout. Participate in a circuit strength-training class, use an elliptical or ride a bike for 30 minutes. Doing so will not only provide a nice change of pace, it also helps to develop different muscles.

Track runs in a diary or journal. Write down the time, date, weather conditions, route, distance and time. When a bad day arrives, which it eventually will, you'll find it helpful to look back on the journal or diary and see how far you have come.

Try to avoid running during periods of high traffic or on busy streets. By running in quieter areas, you take in less exhaust fumes from cars. Look for areas with lots of green space to ensure the lungs stay healthy.

If you find you are bored with running, switch up your route or call on a friend to run with you. There are numerous ways to have fun when you run, and it's just a matter of finding what works for you. Many people find running with a friend helps them progress with their plan.

Chapter 10: Running With Friends

Find a friend to run with. Not only will he or she keep you accountable, you'll find you have someone to keep you motivated when you become discouraged. In addition, boredom is less likely to be an issue when you run with someone else.

It is safer to run with another person. Many runners assume they are safe if they only run during daylight hours. Although it is best to run when it is light outside, you may find you want to run early in the morning or you may not get home until after it is dark. Having a running buddy gives you more time to fit in a workout. In addition, if they have experience, they can assist you with any problems you may encounter or advise you on proper running form.

A running club will be of benefit in this area also. You'll find it easier to locate a running partner when it is convenient to you, if you have a wide group of partners to choose from. Running with different partners will allow you to see different techniques and try various routes, ensuring you don't become bored or discouraged.

A running partner pushes you to go harder and faster. They help you take your running to the next level, so you reach your full potential. Everyone benefits from some fun and friendly competition, and you will do the same. Find a running buddy today and see how you improve rapidly.

Chapter 11: Training Plan

In this chapter you are going to learn how to train to be an avid runner. Before you begin training, here are some key points to keep in mind.

- If you are over the age of 40, not used to regular exercise, or are more than 20 pounds overweight, then you will need to speak with your doctor before you begin. It is best to discuss this with your doctor, especially if you have a health condition.

- You will need to schedule the workouts. You will not find time unless you make the time for them. Put them on your to do lists or in your agenda book. Make time.

- Know that you will have bad days. Everyone has them and it is normal. They will pass fast. Keep in mind that the next run or workout will be better. Just make sure that you keep to the schedule that you have planned in order to ensure you do not fail.

- Do not rush in. Rushing in will lead to injuries and even discourage you. Be sure to be patient and slow. The goal for you is to reach 30 minutes of running.

You are going to be given an eight-week schedule to follow in order to train as a runner. Put the schedule in your agenda book and ensure to follow it till the end. It will ensure that you become the runner you are destined to be.

WEEK ONE:

• **Monday**: Run/Walk – Run for 1 minute, and then walk for 2 minutes. Repeat this 10 times.

• **Tuesday**: Walk – Walk for 30 minutes at a leisurely pace.

• **Wednesday**: Run/Walk – Run for 1 minute, and then walk for 2 minutes. Repeat this 10 times.

• **Thursday**: Walk – Walk for 30 minutes at a leisurely pace.

• **Friday**: Run/Walk – Run for 1 minute, and then walk for 2 minutes. Do this 10 times.

- **Saturday**: Run/Walk – Run for 1 minute, and then walk for 2 minutes. Repeat this 10 times.

- **Sunday**: Rest – Do nothing strenuous in order for your muscles to repair themselves.

WEEK TWO:

- **Monday**: Run/Walk – Run for 2 minutes, and then walk for 1 minute. Repeat this 10 times.

- **Tuesday**: Walk – Walk for 30 minutes at a leisurely pace.

- **Wednesday**: Run/Walk – Run for 3 minutes, and then walk for 1 minute. Repeat this 7 times. Run for the last 2 minutes.

- **Thursday**: Walk – Walk for 30 minutes at a leisurely pace.

- **Friday**: Run/Walk – Run for 4 minutes, and then walk for 1 minute. Repeat this 6 times

- **Saturday**: Run/Walk – Run for 4 minutes, and then walk for 1 minute. Repeat this 6 times

- **Sunday**: Rest – Do nothing to help ensure that your muscles repair themselves.

WEEK THREE:

- **Monday**: Run/Walk – Run for 5 minutes, and then walk for 1 minute. Repeat this 5 times.

- **Tuesday**: Walk – Walk for 30 minutes at a leisurely pace.

- **Wednesday**: Run/Walk – Run for 5 minutes, and then walk for 1 minute. Repeat this 5 times.

- **Thursday**: Walk – Walk for 30 minutes at a leisurely pace.

- **Friday**: Run/Walk – Run for 6 minutes, and then walk for 1 minute. Repeat this 4 times. Run for the next 2 minutes.

- **Saturday**: Run/Walk – Run for 6 minutes, and then walk for 1 minute.

Repeat this 4 times. Run for the last 2 minutes.

• **Sunday**: Rest – Do nothing to allow your body to repair itself.

WEEK FOUR:

• **Monday**: Run/Walk – Run for 8 minutes, and then walk for 1 minute. Repeat it 3 times. Run for 3 minutes.

• **Tuesday**: Walk – Walk at a leisurely pace for 30 minutes.

• **Wednesday**: Run/Walk – Run for 9 minutes, and walk for 1 minutes. Repeat this 3 times.

• **Thursday**: Walk – Walk for 30 minutes at a leisurely pace.

• **Friday**: Run/Walk – Run for 10 minutes, and then walk for 1 minute. Repeat this 2 times, and then run the 8 minutes that are left.

• **Saturday**: Run/Walk – Run for 11 minutes, and then walk for 1 minute. Do this two times. Run the rest of the 8 minutes.

• **Sunday**: Rest – Do nothing in order for your muscles to repair themselves.

WEEK FIVE:

• **Monday**: Run/Walk – Run for 12 minutes, and then walk for 1 minute. Repeat this two times. Run for 4 minutes.

• **Tuesday**: Walk – Walk for 30 minutes at a leisurely pace.

• **Wednesday**: Run/Walk – Run 13 minutes, and then walk for 1 minute. Repeat this 2 times. Run for 2 minutes.

• **Thursday**: Walk – Walk for 30 minutes at a leisurely pace.

• **Friday**: Run/Walk – Run for 14 minutes, walk for 1 minute. Repeat this two times.

• **Saturday**: Run/Walk – Run for 15 minutes, and then walk for 1 minute. Run for 14 minutes.

• **Sunday**: Rest – Do nothing in order to allow your muscles to repair.

WEEK SIX:

- **Monday**: Run/Walk – Run for 16 minutes, and then walk for 1 minute. Run for 13 more minutes.

- **Tuesday**: Walk – Walk for 30 minutes at a leisurely pace.

- **Wednesday**: Run/Walk – Run for 17 minutes, and then walk for 1 minute. Run for 12 minutes.

- **Thursday**: Walk – Walk for 30 minutes leisurely.

- **Friday**: Run/Walk – Run for 18 minutes, and then walk for 1 minute. Run for another 11 minutes.

- **Saturday**: Run/Walk – Run for 19 minute, and then walk for 1 minute. Run for another 10 minutes.

- **Sunday**: Rest – Do nothing in order to allow your muscles to repair.

WEEK SEVEN:

- **Monday**: Run/Walk – Run for 20 minutes, and then walk for 1 minute. Run for the next 9 minutes.

- **Tuesday**: Run/Walk – Run for 20 minutes, and then walk for 1 minute. Run for the next 9 minutes.

- **Wednesday**: Run/Walk – Run for 22 minutes, and then walk for 1 minute. Run for the next 9 minutes.

- **Thursday**: Walk – Walk for 30 minutes at a leisurely pace.

- **Friday**: Run/Walk – Run for 24 minutes, and then walk for 1 minute. Run for the next 7 minutes.

- **Saturday**: Run/Walk – Run for 26 minutes, and then walk for 1 minute. Run for the next 5 minutes.

- **Sunday**: Rest – Do nothing in order for your body to repair itself.

WEEK EIGHT:

- **Monday**: Run/Walk – Run for 27 minutes, and then walk for 1 minute. Run for another 2 minutes.

- **Tuesday**: Run/Walk – Run for 20 minutes, and then walk for 1 minute. Run for another 9 minutes.

- **Wednesday**: Run/Walk – Run for 28 minutes, and then walk for 1 minute. Run for another 1 minute.

- **Thursday**: Walk – Walk for 30 minutes at a leisurely pace.

- **Friday**: Run/Walk – Run for 29 minutes, and then walk for 1 minute.

- **Saturday**: Run/Walk – Run for 30 minutes.

- **Sunday**: Rest – Do nothing to ensure that your body repairs itself.

Chapter 12: Healthy foods for Running

When you run it is important to intake the right nutrients. In this chapter you will learn the best foods that you should intake in order to maintain proper health while working out and running. Not only are these foods great for runners, but if you are in it to win a new body, they will help you lose weight as well. This is what we like to call a "win, win" situation.

White Grapefruit

You should kick start the morning with a white grapefruit in order to get a good healthy dose of some Vitamin C, folate, and potassium. Potassium will keep the muscles from cramping up. After a run in the sun, cut some cold grapefruit and serve it with some mango sorbet for a great treat.

Sweet Potatoes

Sweet potatoes are completely loaded with vitamin A, which is a common food that improves eyesight. They make a wonderful midmorning snack.

Leeks

Iron is extremely important. If you need a healthy boost of running fuel, eat some leeks. They are a great source of iron, vitamin K, and vitamin A. You can pair it with some healthy salmon for an amazingly delicious meal.

Blackberries

Blackberries offer a low calorie snack that is high in antioxidants. Blackberries offer a great amount of fiber, as well as vitamin C. These berries are also full of vitamin K, which also helps to strengthen your bones.

Turnips

Turnips are low in carbohydrates and have a great amount of vitamin C, iron, magnesium, and even calcium. You can plan ahead for the colder days.

Rutabaga

Rutabagas are similar to turnips. They are a great way to intake minerals like magnesium, which helps your body absorb calcium. Rutabagas are able to be cooked, boiled, baked, or even cooked in soup. You can mash them up with other vegetables to make a nutrient packed snack.

Red Grapefruit

Red grapefruits offer high volumes of vitamin C, along with vitamin A and pantothenic acid. The body needs pantothenic acid in order to transform proteins, carbs, and fats to use as energy. Eating a red grapefruit 15-20 minutes before you run, then you will receive a boost of great energy for your workout.

Limes

Limes are extremely low in calories, but extremely high in vitamin C and include some calcium. You can eat these by peeling them or by squeezing the juice on a salad or putting it in some tea. No matter how you intake the lime you will gain benefits from it.

Oranges

Everyone knows that oranges have a high content of vitamin C; however, they do not have to be eaten by themselves. Runners' intake high volumes of vitamin C to ensure a lower level of muscle soreness. Eat them as snacks or put them in another snack or meal.

Winter Squashes

If you need a boost in your immune system, for example, if you are planning on running in inclement weather, then you should eat some winter squash. These are packed with a lot of vitamin A in order to keep you healthy.

Radishes

Radishes have a high content of vitamin C, but they also have a great content of water. They will help you in many ways, as well as keeping you hydrated.

Strawberries

Strawberries are high in vitamin C. Runners should eat plenty of strawberries because they contain anthocyanins, which will repair muscles, as well as fight inflammation. These are great for snacks, and even breakfasts.

Iceberg Lettuce

A large salad is a great meal for lunch or dinner. It offers low calories and a lot of fiber, iron, and folate. It helps runners, and those who would like to lose weight. Therefore, if you are doing the running to shed some pounds, then this is one of the best foods that you can eat.

Lemons

Just like other citrus fruits, lemons are high in vitamin C, but also include thiamin and folate. Runners need thiamin because it helps converts carbs into energy. Do not just add the juice into dishes, put slices of them in meals. Fish is a great meal for lemons.

Tomatoes

Tomatoes are very high in vitamin K, vitamin C, and vitamin A. Those who run reap in the benefits of potassium as well. Add them to almost every meal due to the versatility of this vegetable/fruit. They are definitely considered a super food when it comes to working out and running.

Carrots

Carrots are not only tasty, but are extremely high in vitamin A, as well as carotene and vitamin B6. They improve your immune system and are extremely low in fat. Add these into any meal that you can or eat them raw as a snack.

Cauliflower

The main nutrient in cauliflower is vitamin C. However, it also is packed with folate, pantothenic acid, and vitamin B6. You can eat it raw, steamed, or cooked. Making a soup out of this vegetable is a great and yummy way to ensure the right nutrients for your body.

Scallions

Scallions are high in vitamin K and high in Vitamin A and C. They also offer a lot of folate and manganese. Manganese and folate offers a better digestive system when it comes to breaking down carbs for energy. You can eat them raw with salads or even cook them into meals. They go great with steak, fish, or chicken.

Brussels Sprouts

Brussels sprouts are a great choice due to the high levels of vitamin K and vitamin C. A runner will receive great protein and even fiber along with the other nutrients found in Brussels sprouts. They make a great side dish for steak, chicken, or fish.

Pumpkin

Pumpkin is high in vitamins C and A. They also offer high levels of vitamin E and riboflavin. There are many different recipes that you can make in order to eat pumpkin.

Broccoli

Broccoli offers a high source of vitamin K, vitamin C, folate, as well as manganese. They also contain quercetin, which will help reduce inflammation in the muscles. A great meal idea is broccoli pasta made with whole-wheat noodles.

Arugula

Arugula offers vitamin K, vitamin A, and vitamin C, as well as high levels of magnesium, manganese, calcium, and potassium. You can put it in spring mix or even bake it into some healthy pizza.

Red Bell Peppers

Red bell peppers are an amazing source of vitamin C, vitamin A, as well as vitamin B6. A runner should have vitamin B6 because it will help create hemoglobin, which carries the oxygen in the blood to the muscle tissue. They can be grilled or put in any meal. They are even great on turkey burgers.

Dandelion Greens

Dandelion greens offer a good boost in vitamin K and vitamin A. They are also high in calcium, as well as iron. You can put them into a salad or cook them into other meals or snacks.

Conclusion

Start your running program today. When you see the weight come off, you'll want to run more often. Take it slow for the best results. If you do too much too quickly, you'll do more harm than good. The goal is to build up over time, as this allows you to see the optimal results. If you stick with it, you'll find the weight comes off and you have the motivation to continue. You can do this. All you must do is take the first step.

www.ingramcontent.com/pod-product-compliance
Lightning Source LLC
Chambersburg PA
CBHW071254280526
45788CB00004B/1715